SUMMARY: CURE:

A Journey into the Science of Mind
Over Body
by Jo Merchant |
with BONUS Critics Corner

Authored By

Summary Reads

FREE GIFT SPECIAL REPORT

The Tidiest and Messiest Places on Earth

When summarizing Spark Joy we made a special report about the Tidiest and Messiest Places on Earth! This report is a great supplement to that summary that is all about the virtues of being tidy.

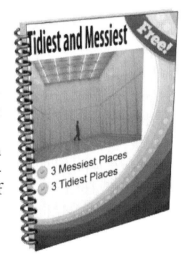

As our **free gift** for being a **SUMMARY READS enthusiast** we are happy to give you a special report about the **3 Most Messy** and the **3 Most Tidy** places on Earth.

Learn about everything from **Garbage Island** to Computer-Chip **Clean Rooms** (and, of course, everything in between).

Get your **free copy** at:

http://sixfigureteen.com/messy

ALSO: We will let you know about future Summary Reads titles so this is **win-win**! Enjoy your **FREE GIFT** and thank you for being part of the **SUMMARY READS** Family!

ISBN-10: 1523928557
ISBN-13: 978-1523928552

DISCLAIMERS

- Absolutely nothing in this volume is meant to constitute legal, financial, or medical advice nor are the opinions presented to be considered expert opinions or the opinions of the author(s) of the original book that we have summarized.
- This volume is **NOT** meant to be a replacement for the original book, we believe our summation, key quotes and highlight analysis will increase interest in the complete book and not detract from it.
- In this volume, each particular detail is presented to the best of our knowledge and understanding of the recent book by Jo Marchant. If you think any of our analysis or summation is inaccurate **please email us** and we will correct it and publish an updated edition after we verify the inconsistency (levelproperty@gmail.com).
- <u>Most importantly</u>: absolutely no portion of this summation volume was written in a Starbucks.

CONTENTS

SUMMARY: CURE – *SINGLE PAGE SUMMARY*

Jo Merchant masterfully explains the power of the mind on the human body in her book CURE.

Jo diligently works to bring story after story in every chapter that enhances the reader's understanding of the power of the mind while evoking emotions for situations that plague this human life.

Through this 12 chapter book shares, in great detail, real stories of human beings that have seen the impact the mind can have on the body. You will be encouraged to utilize your mind in a greater way after reading this book.

CHAPTER SUMMARY 1: FAKING IT: WHY NOTHING WORKS
(SUMMARY, HIGHLIGHTS & BEST QUOTES)

Autism covers a wide spectrum of disorders and is characterized, chiefly, by problems with language and social interaction. All in all it affects about 500,000 children in the U.S. alone.

In 1996, two-year-old Parker Beck from New Hampshire began to slink away from his parents. His laugh left and his smiled ceased. He stopped sleeping through the night and would wake up screaming many times in the middle of the night. Parker was diagnosed with autism.

Parker had a gastrointestinal test called an "endoscopy procedure" performed on him. Though it was an exploratory procedure Parker miraculously got better and better. His smile returned and his playful laugh once again filled the room.

After learning everything one can about the procedure Parker's mother was convinced it was the gut hormone secretin that had brought her little boy back into his old self. As more patients discovered changes once they received secretin a placebo was finally conducted.

30 patients received saline while the other 30 received secretin. Much to the researcher's chagrin there was no connection between secretin and autism. Secretin was a no go for fixing autism. But the fact that plagued the research team was that both groups saw similar improvement in their patients.

Bonnie Anderson fell and broke her back in 2005. She, 75 at the time, remembered how she could no longer golf or enjoy life the way she had in the past. She was offered a surgery called vertebroplasty. This surgery was said to fix 80% of patients. Bonnie was no different, in fact, she felt immensely better the day she left the hospital.

What Bonnie didn't know was that she received a fake surgery. She was part of an experiment to see if the surgery was the reason for success or was it the power of the human mind.

Key Takeaways

At first glance many autistic patients saw dramatic improvement in their behavior with improved eye contact, alertness, and expansion of expressive language.

Vertebroplasty was, at first, considered very effective. Eventually patients would feel better no matter the amount of concrete placed in their spine or even if the conrete was placed in the wrong location. This led doctors at the Mayo Clinic to perform a placebo like test that Bonnie, unknowingly, was a part of.

YOU DECIDE: @SummaryReads

CHAPTER SUMMARY 2: A DEVIANT IDEA: WHEN MEANING IS EVERYTHING
(SUMMARY, HIGHLIGHTS & BEST QUOTES)

Linda Buonanno suffers from Irritable Bowel Syndrome. It has taken away her life. She has been reduced to visiting new places with Google Earth, as she must sit near a bathroom at all times.

As Lisa looked for relief she discovered a bold medical test group ran by Dr. Ted Kaptchuck, a professor at Harvard Medical School in Boston. This test group tested the effects of a placebo pill.

Dr. Kaptchuck started his education interested in Eastern religions and philosophies. He attended medical school in China and came back to the States and opened up an acupuncture clinic in Cambridge. He began to see dramatic cures for patients many times before any treatment had taken place. He began to realize all it took was a conversation between he and the patient where he could give them hope.

Dr. Kaptchuck compared the effectiveness of two different kinds of placebo - fake acupuncture and a fake pill. Though conventional wisdom would say a trial testing nothing against nothing should yield no results, Dr. Kaptchuck saw something entirely different. The placebo acupuncture was more effective for reducing the patients' pain, whereas the placebo pill worked better for helping them to sleep.

Dan Moerman, University of Michigan anthropologist, believes that the active ingredient in a placebo is meaning. His goal is to change the name placebo to the meaning response, but it is not catching on.

Lisa Buonanno started this trial, knowing it was a placebo, and started feeling much better in three days. For the three weeks of the trial Lisa found life again. Yet, three days after the trial ended her IBS came back and she was house ridden one more time.

Key Takeaways

Dr. Kaptchuck saw patients with all sorts of conditions at his acupuncture clinic. Most of these conditions were chronic complaints from pain to digestive, urinary and respiratory problems.

One key to remember is that placebo trial results vary greatly in different parts of the world. For a particular ulcer medicine Denmark saw 59% positive reaction for the placebo while Brazil say just 7%.

The IBS trial published in 2010 found that those patients that knowingly took the placebo did significantly better than those who received no treatment.

YOU DECIDE: @SummaryReads:

CHAPTER SUMMARY 3: PAVLOV'S POWER: HOW TO TRAIN YOUR IMMUNE SYSTEM
(SUMMARY, HIGHLIGHTS & BEST QUOTES)

Karl-Heinz is a retired psychologist from Germany. For years he was on dialysis until he received a kidney transplant. Now he takes pills to suppress his immune system every day for the rest of his life.

Along with these pills he has started taking a new pill, drinking a green liquid, and listening to the Johnny Cash song *Help Me*. This new part of his regiment is a trial based upon the placebo effect. The hope is that it will train his immune system to not need the other medication and give him more freedom in his life.

This study Karl is submitting himself too is based upon the experiments of Ivan Pavlov. Pavlov famously trained dogs with stimuli such as light or a bell. In the same way researchers hope to train the body to react positively to placebos in order to change the body's reaction to disease.

One Pavlov like research experiment involved rats. These rats were given sweet water and an injection of cytoxan. Cytoxan, deadly in high injections, is an ingredient that made the rats sick to the stomach. The rats wouldn't drink the sweet water with no injection because they associated the sweet water with the cytoxan and the illness that followed.

Even stranger the researchers force-fed the rats sweet water with no cytoxan. One by one the rats died because their immune system remembered the illness and weakened itself to where the cytoxan killed them.

Key Takeaways

Placebos can create biological changes in the body, yet, most influence symptoms but cannot change the underlying disease.

If a person is giving a medicine with active healing ingredients and then take placebos they have a 95-100% response rate, because their body expects to get better.

YOU DECIDE: **@SummaryReads:**

CHAPTER SUMMARY 4: FIGHTING FATIGUE: THE ULTIMATE PRISON BREAK

(SUMMARY, HIGHLIGHTS & BEST QUOTES)

No one had climbed Mt. Everest before without the aide of oxygen. However, Reinhold Messner and Peter Habeler were determined to climb the world's tallest peak without any additional oxygen. The reached the top when no one thought the body could operate in that altitude without additional oxygen.

Tim Noakes, a sports physiologist at the University of Cape Town, South Africa, carried out a study in the 1980s that showed that runners weren't collapsing in marathons from dehydration, rather, from drinking too many liquids. In the U.S. at the time the official advice to runners suggested 50 ounces of liquids an hour during a run. Noakes determined this was poisoning them.

Noakes suggests that we can push our brain farther. He believes our brain has a governor that convinces the body it has nothing left and to quit. Retraining that part of the brain or ignoring it will show that you can go farther and push harder. Your body does have something left.

Key Takeaways

A 2009 study of climbers ascending into Everest found that near the summit the oxygen content of their blood plummeted to just three quarters of normal levels. However, blood levels at 23,300 feet and lower showed no oxygen changed from sea level. The findings showed that whatever plagued climbers and forced them to stop before 23,300 feet was something different than lack of oxygen.

Noakes discovered that race officials in the States were being influenced by sports drink companies and it wasn't until the 2002 Boston Marathon, where 13% of participants suffered water intoxication, including the death of one runner, that led to a change in the official advice of liquid consumption.

YOU DECIDE: @SummaryReads:

CHAPTER SUMMARY 5: IN A TRANCE: IMAGINE YOUR GUT AS A RIVER
(SUMMARY, HIGHLIGHTS & BEST QUOTES)

Emma, 21, holds a piping hot water bottle on her side. Though her skin is raw and red from the heat she refuses to let it go. To the casual observer she is a woman giving birth, except there is no baby and she goes through this every day.

Fraser, in his late forties, has permanent and uncontrollable diarrhea. He has stood with his back against the wall protecting his soiled jeans from the sight of those at a party. He stands with his back to them until the last person leaves the party.

Emma and Fraser, as well as many others, suffer from irritable bowel syndrome (IBS). Around 15% of people worldwide suffer from IBS and most conventional treatments are not effective.

To make matters worse there appears to be nothing wrong with the gut and very few people understand how real IBS is to those afflicted. Often these patients find a doctor that tells them this is functional and the patient should deal with it.

Dr. Peter Whorwell is a gastroenterologist and specializes in helping people plagued with IBS. He started using hypnotics as a tool to relax the gut. He felt if it helped relax muscles then it may work on the gut as well.

A few weeks after going to Dr. Whorwell patients began noticing a relaxation in their gut that helps alleviate many symptoms of IBS. Dr. Whorwell focuses the patient on how eating feels and how it goes into your stomach.

In the end the goal is that you control your IBS your IBS does not control you. The brain and the gut are intricately connected. There is a constant stream of communication between the two. These are as simple as our stomach telling us we are hungry to warning us that we've eaten something poisonous and need to vomit.

Key Takeaways

Hypnotics got its medically bad name from a doctor in the 18th century that would wave his hands around a patient to get their animal life flow flowing the proper way. He was widely discredited and thus, hypnotics became something of an albatross to the rest of the medical field.

YOU DECIDE: @SummaryReads:

CHAPTER SUMMARY 6: RETHINKING PAIN: INTO THE ICE CANYON
(SUMMARY, HIGHLIGHTS & BEST QUOTES)

In 2008, Lieutenant Sam Brown was hit with an IED roadside bomb in Kandahar, Afghanistan. He suffered third degree burns over most of his body. The recovery and healing is the most agonizing part of third degree burns. Eventually, Brown was asked if he wanted to take part in a pioneering research trial.

For years new pain medication has come to the market. Doctors now have patients on pain medication for months or years. Coming off these drugs has horrible side effects as patients suffer from anxiety, hypersensitivity, and even addiction.

Key Takeaways

A new wave of distraction has begun to be researched, visual imagery. Patients are taken to a secure and happy place through images and sounds while pain in inflicted and the results have shown that the experience is more pleasant than without the visual imagery distracting them.

YOU DECIDE: **@SummaryReads:**

CHAPTER SUMMARY 7: TALK TO ME: WHY CARING MATTERS

(SUMMARY, HIGHLIGHTS & BEST QUOTES)

91% of women that give birth to a child say it is the most intense pain they have ever felt, even with pain-killing drugs. Though first world countries have very low death rates for the mothers and babies this is still a traumatic event.

A study in 2012 revealed that women who have one-to-one continuous support, not nurses and midwives that go off shift, through labor are less likely to need a C-section or instrumental birth.

Emotional support from someone the woman trusts can reduce fear and help the mother feel more in control. Research also shows that easing anxiety can influence the physical progress of labor directly.

Key Takeaways

Continuous care's strongest benefits come from developing countries where women are frightened or uneducated about labor. A study found in the U.S. and Canada that continuous care didn't reduce the rate of interventions at all.

YOU DECIDE: **@SummaryReads:**

CHAPTER SUMMARY 8: FIGHT OR FLIGHT: THOUGHTS THAT KILL

(SUMMARY, HIGHLIGHTS & BEST QUOTES)

Robert Kloner, a Los Angeles cardiologist, remembers the LA earthquake of 1994. As he was awakened by the quake he felt like his heart was going to beat out of his chest or even stop altogether. Few demonstrations of the mind's effects on the body are as dramatic as sheer terror.

Kloner later discovered that dozens of people died in the quake with no real injuries other than thinking they were going to die. The emergency response to terror our body initiates is known as fight or flight.

Unlike other mammals humans learn from our mistakes and work toward the future. As a zebra calms down after running away from a lion a human will go over the turns and the close calls in their mind over and over.

Chronic stress will, in the long run, lead to physical problems. One research team in the UK discovered that employees with the most stressful jobs tend to live shorter life spans than those with less stress in their lives. Bottom line is that stress can play a major role on all aspects of our body.

Key Takeaways

For two weeks leading to the earthquake an average of 73 people died everyday from heart attacks; 125 died on the day of the earthquake. This suggests that 50 people's hearts failed as a direct consequence of the disaster.

YOU DECIDE: @SummaryReads

CHAPTER SUMMARY 9: ENJOY THE MOMENT: HOW TO CHANGE YOUR BRAIN

(SUMMARY, HIGHLIGHTS & BEST QUOTES)

In the last decade a new generation of brain imaging studies, along with clinical trials, has put meditation on the scientific map. These studies have started showing that meditation can have hard physical effects on our brains and bodies.

Researchers believe they have found a link to our minds and meditation. They state that training the mind to be more aware of current surroundings can reduce stress and anxiety in your daily routine.

What happens for people not meditating, researchers say, one notices the mental world and not the current world. In other words as you are completing a task your mind is already focused on the next big task you must complete, this adds stress.

Negative thoughts trigger negative responses in the body. As you are preparing for bed one night you and are thinking about the big meeting tomorrow at the office you can start feeling unneeded stress because you are worrying about something you cannot control at the time.

Mindfulness meditation aims to stop this stress over future or past events from happening. It forces you to become more aware of your own thoughts and to take a step back and realize that a negative or stressful notion doesn't necessarily represent reality.

Mindfulness meditation reminds us that we do not have

to respond emotionally to what is cruising the interstate of our minds.

Key Takeaways

There are hundreds of ways to meditate but mindfulness is a meditation technique that is taking the United States by storm. Mindfulness involves being aware of your own thoughts and surroundings.

The more stressed we feel, the more likely we are to come up with negative thoughts.

YOU DECIDE: **@SummaryReads:**

CHAPTER SUMMARY 10: FOUNTAIN OF YOUTH: THE SECRET POWER OF FRIENDS

(SUMMARY, HIGHLIGHTS & BEST QUOTES)

The Nicoya peninsula in northwestern Costa Rica has created an interesting case study in the power of human connection. In general, people live longest in the world's richest countries, this is not the case for the Nicoyans.

Nicoyans are known to live longer and have younger looking cells, under a microscope, than almost any other people group in the world. But this isn't about money, in fact, Costa Rica has a GDP of about 1/5 of the United States and the Nicoya peninsula is one of the poorest regions in Costa Rica.

Nicoyans have active lifestyles in old age, strong religious faith, lack of electricity forces them to go to bed earlier, and they drink calcium-rich water. All these have a positive affect on the human body.

But the key determining factor is that Nicoyans are less likely to live alone than other Costa Ricans. Nicoyans have a strong family bond so much so that they see their children an average of once a week.

Loneliness has a tremendous impact on the human body. The more isolated and lonely one feels the more likely they are to live shorter lives and struggle with health.

Research even shows that people that get sick and have a strong group of people connected to them have a stronger chance to win the battle with illness than those that are more isolated.

Key Takeaways

The impact of loneliness depends not on how many physical contacts we have but how isolated we feel.

YOU DECIDE: **@SummaryReads:**

CHAPTER SUMMARY 11: GOING ELECTRIC: NERVES THAT CURE
(SUMMARY, HIGHLIGHTS & BEST QUOTES)

A new practice for those that struggle with heart rate variability (HRV) has seen tremendous results. The practice is called HRV biofeedback and it uses the heart rate monitor and a computer display to help patients get their heart rate to run into a smooth curve.

Proponents claim that this practice has a wide range of benefits such as:

- Strengthening our hearts
- Reducing stress
- Increased happiness
- Decreased stress levels

The story of a badly burned 11-month-old girl named Janice, who died a month later from complications, led Dr. Kevin Tracey to research sepsis and figure out how to save his next patients life. His research led him to the same structure in the body that HRV biofeedback targeted: the vagus nerve.

Key Takeaways

There are several processes in the body that cause our heart rate to fluctuate. One of these is baroreflex and it is a reflex controlled by the nervous system.

YOU DECIDE: @SummaryReads

CHAPTER SUMMARY 12: LOOKING FOR GOD: THE REAL MIRACLE OF THE LOURDES

(SUMMARY, HIGHLIGHTS & BEST QUOTES)

In 1858 a little girl in France was said to have heard the Virgin Mary speaking to her and when she finished water poured out from the area she spoke. This water is said to have healing power and is called the Lourdes. In fact the Lourdes is a major pilgrimage point for Catholics now.

Science makes very little room for God. Richard Dawkins and Stephen Hawking have written entire books dedicated to eradicating the need for God. This makes the Lourdes a very interesting study as God and science meet.

Much recent research concludes that being religious leads to better emotional or psychological health. In fact, an increasing amount of studies are now claiming physical benefits as well.

One study asked half the group to pick a phrase for meditation such as "God is love" or "God is peace" while the other half picked phrases such as "I am happy" or "grass is green." The volunteers meditated for 20 minutes a day for two weeks then the researchers tested their pain tolerance. Those in spiritual meditation were able to hold their hands in ice cold water for nearly twice as long as those not in the spiritual group.

In another study of 83 migraine sufferers, those who practiced spiritual meditation for a month had fewer headaches and greater pain tolerance than those that practiced secular meditation. The results brought the researchers to this decision: content counts.

These small studies need additional research to hold up but there is a growing sense of understanding that a spiritual perspective may help to reduce the emotional impact of pain by placing it in the larger picture.

Key Takeaways

Since 1858 more than 7,000 people have reported themselves as miracles at the Lourdes. Through research and the decision of a bishop 69 of them have been stamped as miracles.

YOU DECIDE: @SummaryReads

Bonus Feature: Critics Corner

At Summary Reads we always enjoy summarizing best-sellers for those with not enough time read all the best-sellers coming out or just want to get a taste before deciding to get a full version (which is always much more expensive.)

We think New York Times Book Review said it very well in its review of the book:

Ms. Marchant writes well, which is never a guarantee in this genre... Second, [she] has chosen very moving characters to show us the importance of the research... and she has an equal flair for finding inspirational figures... the studies are irresistible, and they come in an almost infinite variety

Even readers that gave it a lukewarm review just comment that their expectations were higher and not that the book was not written well or didn't have value. The worst review we could find stated this:

"Although I liked a lot of the book, it does seem a little too clinical in many aspects "

FURTHER READING

Are you ready to quickly absorb the main points and highlights of the next best seller? Check out the other great summaries from *Summary Reads*:

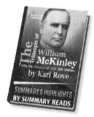

■ Karl Rove's latest book, ***The Triumph of William McKinley: Why the Election of 1896 Still Matters*** is a great read, but it is a LONG book. We have already read it and summarized it for you so pick up a copy and enjoy:

http://amzn.com/B018YOPOJY

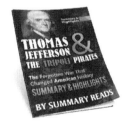

■ Brian Kilmeade's latest best-seller, ***Thomas Jefferson and the Tripoli Pirates,*** is a fascinating story about a forgotten war. Get the summary today:

http://amzn.com/B018B8FFWK

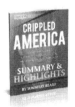

■ Crippled America is Trump's latest book and we have the top summary on the market:

http://amzn.com/B017QT0IMM

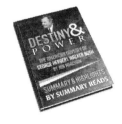

■ The over 900 page best-seller ***Destiny and Power*** is a great book but not everyone has the time for the whole book. Check out our summary and save hours: http://amzn.com/B019D70GI6

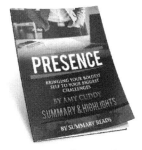

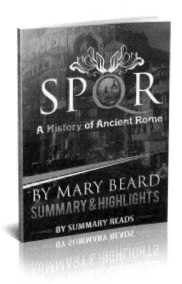

IF YOU LIKED this summary then you will **LOVE** our summary of **"Presence**: Bringing Your **Boldest Self** to Your Biggest Challenges" by **Amy Cuddy**…

Learn how **small changes** in your daily habits can have HUGE **positive effects** on your life!
http://amzn.com/B01A14U1W6

Last but **DEFINITELY NOT LEAST** is our best-seller summary of Mary Beard's *SPQR: A History of Ancient Rome*.

Get your copy today:
http://amzn.com/B018MANYA2

FREE GIFT SPECIAL REPORT
The 10 Strange Deaths of Vladimir Putin

A major part of **Trump's foreign policy** message is that he will be able to work together with the Russian head-of-state Vladimir Putin, but what kind of man is Mr. Putin?

As our **free gift** for being a **SUMMARY READS** enthusiast we are happy to give you a special report about some of the mysterious and <u>strange deaths</u> that have befallen Mr. Putin's enemies.

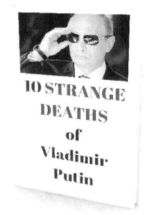

Plane crashes, multiple stab wounds and radioactive sushi are just a few of the misfortunes that have befallen those who opposed the Russian President.

Get your free copy at:

http://sixfigureteen.com/summaryreads

<u>ALSO</u>: We will let you know about future Summary Reads titles so this is win-win! Enjoy your FREE GIFT and thank you for being part of the SUMMARY READS Family!

FREE GIFT SPECIAL REPORT

The Tidiest and Messiest Places on Earth

When summarizing Spark Joy we made a special report about the Tidiest and Messiest Places on Earth! This report is a great supplement to that summary that is all about the virtues of being tidy.

As our **free gift** for being a **SUMMARY READS enthusiast** we are happy to give you a special report about the **3 Most Messy** and the **3 Most Tidy** places on Earth.

Learn about everything from **Garbage Island** to Computer-Chip **Clean Rooms** (and, of course, everything in between).

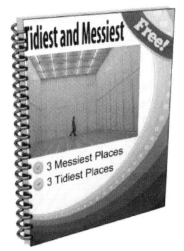

Get your **free copy** at:

http://sixfigureteen.com/messy

<u>ALSO</u>: We will let you know about future Summary Reads titles so this is **win-win**! Enjoy your **FREE GIFT** and thank you for being part of the **SUMMARY READS** Family!

Made in the USA
Las Vegas, NV
08 January 2024